MEDITERRANEAN DIET COOKBOOK

Mediterranean Diet Guide for Beginners Recipes for Weight Loss and Healthy Eating, Delicious Recipes & Desserts and 7 Tips for Weight Loss

(The Ultimate Beginners Mediterranean Diet Cookbook)

Somerville Jacques

Published by Jason Thawne Publishing House

© Somerville Jacques

Mediterranean Diet cookbook: Mediterranean Diet Guide for Beginners Recipes for Weight Loss and Healthy Eating, Delicious Recipes & Desserts and 7 Tips for Weight Loss

(The Ultimate Beginners Mediterranean Diet Cookbook)

All Rights Reserved

ISBN 978-1-989749-95-1

This document is geared towards providing exact and reliable information in regards to the topic and issue covered. The publication is sold with the idea that the publisher isn't required to render accounting, officially permitted, or otherwise, qualified services. If advice is necessary, legal or even professional, a practiced individual in the profession should be ordered.

- From a Declaration of Principles which was accepted and approved equally by a Committee of the American Bar Association and a Committee of Publishers and Associations.

In no way is it legal to reproduce, duplicate, or even transmit any part of this document in either electronic means or in printed format. Recording of this publication is strictly prohibited and any storage of this document isn't allowed unless with proper written permission from the publisher. All rights reserved.

The information provided herein is stated to be truthful and consistent, in that any liability, in terms of inattention or otherwise, by any usage or abuse of any policies, processes, or directions contained within is the solitary and also utter responsibility of the recipient reader. Under no circumstances will any legal responsibility or blame be held against the publisher for any reparation, damages, or monetary loss due to the information herein, either directly or indirectly.

Respective authors own all copyrights not held by the publisher.

The information herein is offered for just informational purposes solely, and is universal as so. The presentation of the information is without contract or any type of guarantee assurance.

The trademarks that are used are without any consent, and also the publication of the trademark is without permission or backing by the trademark owner. All trademarks and brands within this book are for clarifying purposes only and are the owned by the owners themselves, not affiliated with this document.

TABLE OF CONTENTS

Part 1 1

Introduction 2

Chapter 1 – Why Go Mediterranean 3

Chapter 2 – Breakfast Options 7

The Classic Greek Salad Recipe 7

Omelet With Salmon And Asparagus 8

Baked Falafel 9

Toast With Cheese, Fruit And Nuts 11

Creamy Mediterranean Paninis 11

Granola With Fruit And Nuts 12

Basic Mediterranean Fish (Halibut) 13

Mediterranean Breakfast Smoothie 14

Mustard Trout And Lady Apples 14

Oatmeal With Fruit And Nuts 16

Mediterranean Chicken Wrap 17

Mediterranean Feta And Eggplant Dip 18

Chapter 3 – Lunch Options 20

Chopped Salad With Chicken – Greek Style 20

Mediterranean Tuna Salad 21

Zucchini And Goat Cheese Frittata 22

Mediterranean Pasta Salad 24

Rhubarb Lentil Soup	25
Mediterranean Chicken Stew	27
Kale & White Bean Soup With Sausage	28
Cheesy Chive Potatoes	30
Chickpea Salad	32
Couscous And Dried Cherries Salad	33
Mediterranean Watermelon Salad	34
Chapter 4 – Dinner Options	36
Curry Rubbed Salmon With Napa Slaw	36
Crisp Lamb Lettuce Wraps	38
Greek Lamb Chops	39
Chicken Kebabs	40
Seared Mediterranean Tuna Steaks	41
Greek Dinner Salad	43
Super-Fast Kofte	44
Greek Feta Burgers	46
Lemon Basil Shrimp And Pasta	47
Moussaka	48
Dirty Potatoes	50
Chopped Greek Chicken Salad	51
Chapter 5 – Snacks And Other Sides	53
Marinated Olives Plus Feta	53

Mediterranean Pick Me Up Snack	54
Quick Mediterranean Dip	55
Creamy Artichoke Dip	56
Potato Croquettes With Parmesan	57
Mediterranean Hummus	58
Pine Nuts And Spinach Orzo	59
Simple Mediterranean Layered Dip	61
Basic Greek Salad	62
Creamy Mediterranean Dip	63
Tzatziki	64
5 Layer Greek Dip	65
8 Layer Mediterranean Dip	66
Quick Mediterranean Egg Snack	67
Conclusion	68
Part 2	69
Breakfast Recipes	70
Creamy Date Smoothie	70
Toast With Avocado	71
Fruity Yogurt Parfait	73
Couscous With Dried Fruit	75
Mixed Veggie Omelet	77
Scrambled Eggs With Veggies	79

Cheesy Veggie Muffins 81

Cheesy Zucchini Frittata 83

Oats Pancakes 85

Yogurt Crepes 87

Lunch Recipes 89

Cucumber & Olives Salad 90

Chickpeas & Veggie Gazpacho 91

Lamb Filled Pita With Yogurt Sauce 93

Chickpea Patties 95

Stuffed Tomatoes 98

Veggie Pizza 100

Chicken & Veggie Kebabs 102

Herbed Pasta With Tomatoes 105

Couscous With Cauliflower & Dates 106

Prawns With Garlic Sauce 109

Dinner Recipes 111

Beans & Spinach Soup 111

Seafood Stew 114

Salmon With Veggies 116

Mussels In Wine & Tomato Sauce 118

Lamb Chops With Herbed Pistachios 120

Lamb Kofta With Spicy Yogurt Sauce 122

Chicken With Capers Sauce 125

Steak With Yogurt Sauce 127

Pasta With Veggies 130

Conclusion 133

About The Author 133

Part 1

Introduction

I want to thank you and congratulate you for downloading the book, World's Healthiest Diets – Mediterranean Diet: 50 Quick, Easy and Delicious Mediterranean Diet Recipes to Lose Weight and Be Healthy.

This book contains recipes that have helped people to lose weight. It provides you with a wide array of options for breakfast, lunch, dinners, and snacks. Dips and other side dishes have also been included to help enhance the flavors of any meal.

The average preparation time of these recipes are from 5 to 15 minutes. You will have more time enjoying most of the meals than preparing them. Each of the recipes included here are packed with the distinct flavors of the Mediterranean.

Enjoy the dishes and enjoy their health benefits.

Thanks again for downloading this book!

Chapter 1 – Why Go Mediterranean

A lot of studies have been done on the many diets available including the Mediterranean Diet. Many diet and fitness experts classify this diet as a balanced type of diet. They basically place it in the same class as the Mayo Clinic Diet, DASH Diet, and the Vegetarian Diet.

Some studies that investigated the Mediterranean Diet say it has the capability to induce weight loss. Some studies indicate that it promotes brain and heart health. There some indications that it may help in cancer and diabetes prevention or control.

The Hype – Mixing Wheat with the Tares

Unfortunately, a lot of hype has also been included whenever marketers try to convince people to try the diet. The claims go from simple weight loss and get blown up to preventing a lot of chronic diseases. Of course, there are studies that suggest these possibilities but in reality, their research is still not 100% there.

The Hip and Fit Mediterranean

One of the reasons why people have become interested in the Mediterranean diet is the overall fitness observed among the people who live along the coast of the Mediterranean Sea. A lot of people have the opinion that the Mediterranean folks live longer and don't suffer as much of the health problems in other countries such as the US.

Of course, people investigated their peculiarities including their diet. The secret of these hip and happy people is not only found in their diet but also in the active lifestyles they live. If you really want to live by Mediterranean standards, then you should not only eat what they eat; you should also live how they live.

Does It Really Help People Lose Weight?

As stated earlier, the research on this area of interest isn't 100 percent just yet. But there are studies as early as 2008 that show that this diet can create a calorie deficit in people. What we know so far is that this diet can at least help you shed some pounds. Its overall efficiency at reducing a lot of weight is still subjective to each person who follows the diet.

Cardiovascular and Other Health Benefits

The Mediterranean Diet is believed to help reduce the risk of cardiovascular diseases. It has been demonstrated that it can help reduce bad cholesterol and reduce one's blood pressure. However, it should also be pointed out that its effects are moderately provided. It's not an instant solution for people who are suffering from the above mentioned health conditions.

How Safe Is It?

There are no known health risks if people try this diet. The diet basically espouses the use of olive oil as its primary source of oil. The centerpiece of every recipe is fruits and veggies. It also provides a healthy helping of both bread and pasta.

The recipes in this diet may include meat but when it does, they are usually in small portions. Mediterranean dinners usually include at least a glass of red wine. For food flavor, you will usually make use of herbs such as basil, mint, garlic, rosemary, and lemon. Salt is used sparingly.

Chapter 2 – Breakfast Options

The Classic Greek Salad Recipe

Ingredients:

oregano leaves (handful)

5 cucumbers (cucumber)

1 cup olive oil

1 cup cherry tomatoes (chopped)

1 small red onion

grated zest and juice of 1 lemon

1 tsp. honey

1 tsp. dried oregano

1 cup kalamata olives

kosher salt

¼ cup red wine vinegar

freshly ground pepper

4 oz. feta cheese

Instructions:

Slice red onion. Soak in salted water. Combine lemon zest, half a teaspoon of salt, vinegar, dried oregano, honey, ¼ tsp. pepper, and lemon juice. Whisk mixture. Add olive oil slowly until everything is blended well. Toss in tomatoes and olives (halved and pitted).

Slice cucumbers into lengthwise pieces. Add them to the mixture. Add chopped tomatoes to the salad mixture. Drain the salt water from onions. Toss it with the rest of the ingredients.

Drain and slice feta into even rectangles. Use oregano and cheese as toppings. Season your salad with pepper. As a final touch drizzle oil on salad.

Omelet with Salmon and Asparagus

Ingredients:

4 oz. salmon

2 tbsp. onion (diced)

½ tsp. canola oil

¼ tsp. lemon juice

½ tbsp. parsley

2 asparagus spears (steamed)

1 tsp. low fat milk

2 eggs

Instructions:

Sauté onions over medium heat. Add garlic, asparagus, and lemon juice. Beat the eggs in a bowl. Add milk and parsley. Add salt, pepper, dill and chives to the sautéed onions. Add eggs to vegetable mix and let it set for one minute. Add salmon bring heat to low. Cook eggs for three minutes. Fold omelet in half then cook for one minute. Serve.

Baked Falafel

Ingredients:

1 (15 ounce) can garbanzo beans, rinsed and drained

1/4 cup chopped fresh parsley

1/4 cup chopped onion

1/4 tsp. ground coriander

1 tbsp. all-purpose flour

3 cloves garlic (minced)

1/4 tsp. salt

1/4 teaspoon baking soda

1 tsp. ground cumin

1 beaten egg

2 tsps. olive oil

Instructions:

Wrap onion in cheese cloth and then squeeze out its moisture. Set aside. Mix salt, garlic, cumin, coriander, garbanzo beans, parsley, and baking soda in a food processor. Add onion to mixture and put in a bowl. Stir in flour and egg. Shape mixture into patties. Let them stand for 15 minutes.

Preheat an oven to 400 degrees Fahrenheit. Heat olive oil over medium-high heat. Place the patties in the skillet. Cook until golden brown. Place skillet in oven and bake for 10 minutes. Serve.

Toast with Cheese, Fruit and Nuts

Ingredients:

¾ oz. low calorie cheese

½ tsp. walnuts (chopped)

½ pear (peeled, cored, and sliced)

1 slice whole grain bread

Instructions:

Toast the bread. Spread with cheese. Top with the pear and nuts.

Creamy Mediterranean Paninis

Ingredients:

1 seven oz. jar of roasted red peppers (drained and sliced)

2 tablespoons finely chopped oil-cured black olives

¼ cup chopped fresh basil leaves

8 slices rustic whole grain bread

1 small zucchini (sliced thinly)

4 slices provolone cheese

Instructions:

Combine ¼ cup mayonnaise dressing with olive oil, basil, and olives. Evenly this mixture on bread slices. Layer it with peppers, provolone, bacon, and zucchini. Top with other bread slices. Spread mayonnaise mixture on the outside. Cook over medium heat until golden brown.

Granola with Fruit and Nuts

Ingredients:

¼ medium apple, cored, peeled and diced

½ cup low fat granola

1 tsp. walnuts (chopped)

½ cup low fat or fat free milk

¼ banana, sliced and peeled

Instructions:

Mix granola and milk. Top with walnuts, banana, and apple.

Basic Mediterranean Fish (Halibut)

Ingredients:

4 (6 ounce) halibut fillets

1 (5 ounce) jar pitted kalamata olives

1 tablespoon Greek seasoning

1 onion (chopped)

1 tbsp. lemon juice

salt

pepper

¼ cup capers

1 large tomato (chopped)

¼ cup olive oil

Instructions:

Preheat oven to 350 degrees Fahrenheit. Put halibut fillets on aluminum foil sheet. Season them with Greek seasoning. Combine onion, tomato, capers, olives, olive oil, salt, pepper, and lemon juice. Spoon the tomato mixture on halibut. Seal all edges of foil. Place on a baking sheet. Bake in oven for 30 to 40 minutes.

Mediterranean Breakfast Smoothie

Ingredients:

½ tbsp. flaxseed

2 oz. pure pomegranate juice

½ small banana

½ cup mixed berries

4 ice cubes

¼ cup apple juice

Instructions:

In a Blender, bend ice cubes, fruits, juices, and flax seed. Use high setting. Blend until smooth. Serve.

Mustard Trout and Lady Apples

Ingredients:

1 shallot (minced)

1 tbsp. capers

1 cup apple cider

1 tsp. fresh thyme (chopped)

1 tbsp. Dijon mustard

2 tsp. light-brown sugar

3 tbsp. plain bread crumbs

2 tbsp. olive oil

4 lady apples (lengthwise pieces, cored)

coarse salt and ground pepper

8 trout fillets

1 tbsp. unsalted butter (melted)

Instructions:

Preheat oven to 375 degrees Fahrenheit. Mix thyme, bread crumbs, and shallot. Season with salt and pepper. Add butter. Give it a light toss.

Place apple pieces cut-side up baking dish. Sprinkle sugar on top. Top them with bread-crumb mixture. Pour cider around apples. Cover and bake for half an hour. Uncover and bake 20 minutes more.

Turn oven to broil. Place rack 4 inches from heat. Pat trout fillets with paper towels. Season them with salt and pepper. Brush a baking sheet with 1 tbsp. oil. Place trout skin-side up on baking sheet. Brush trout skin with remaining oil. Broil 6 minutes. Reheat apples on shelf underneath trout for 1 to 2 minutes.

Whisk together mustard, ¾ cup cider, and capers. Cook over medium-high heat. Reduce mixture to sauce consistency. Place a pair of halibut fillets side by side on plates. Spoon the juices around fish fillets. Add two apple halves next to fillets. Garnish with thyme.

Oatmeal with Fruit and Nuts

Ingredients:

½ cup oats

1 tsp. sunflower seeds

1 tsp. almonds (sliced)

¼ mango (diced)

½ apple (diced)

1 cup fat free milk

Instructions:

Combine oats and milk in a microwaveable bowl. Microwave the mixture on high setting for a total of two minutes. Mix in almonds and sunflower seeds. Top with mango and apple.

Mediterranean Chicken Wrap

Ingredients:

2 cans artichoke hearts (thinly sliced)

1 chicken cutlet (3 ounces)

¼ cup mixed baby greens

Coarse salt and ground pepper

½ small tomato (thinly sliced)

1 whole-wheat wrap

1 tbsp. olive tapenade

Instructions:

Season the chicken with salt and pepper. Broil until opaque throughout. Let cool. Spread olive tapenade on bottom of wheat wrap. Layer it with baby greens, tomato, artichoke hearts, and chicken. Season with salt and pepper. Fold to seal.

Mediterranean Feta and Eggplant Dip

Ingredients:

1 small chili pepper

1 regular size eggplant

¼ tsp. salt

¼ tsp. cayenne pepper

1 tbsp. finely chopped flat-leaf parsley

2 tbsp. chopped fresh basil

½ cup red onion

¼ cup olive oil

2 tbsp. of fresh squeezed lemon juice

½ cup feta cheese (grated)

1 red bell pepper (diced)

Instructions:

Get some foil and use it to line a baking pan. Position the rack about half a foot above the oven's fire. Preheat broiler.

Poke holes on the eggplant to serve as vents. Place it in the pan. Broil until well-done. Set aside to cool.

Scrape eggplant flesh into bowl and add lemon juice. Toss. Add oil. Stir well. Chop onion and stir it in. Add feta cheese, parsley, chili pepper, basil, salt, cayenne, and bell pepper. Serve.

Chapter 3 – Lunch Options

Chopped Salad with Chicken – Greek Style

Ingredients:

6 cups chopped romaine lettuce

1/3 cup red-wine vinegar

½ cup feta cheese

2 tbsp. olive oil

1 medium cucumber (chopped)

1 tbsp. chopped fresh dill

2 ½ cups chopped cooked chicken breast

½ cup sliced ripe black olives

1 tsp. garlic powder

2 medium tomatoes (chopped)

¼ tsp. salt

½ cup red onion (chopped)

¼ tsp. freshly ground pepper

Instructions:

Whisk garlic powder, salt, oil, dill, vinegar, and pepper. Add lettuce, olives cucumber, onion, chicken, tomatoes, and crumbled feta. Toss ingredients.

Mediterranean Tuna Salad

Ingredients:

1 large can albacore tuna (drained)

1 celery stalk (diced), leaves reserved

1 strip (1 1/2 inches) lemon zest, thinly sliced

3 tbsp. fresh lemon juice

3 tbsp. almonds

1 tbsp. and 2 tsp. olive oil

2 tbsp. drained brine-packed capers (chopped)

coarse salt

freshly ground pepper

¼ cup dill sprigs

8 ounces mixed salad greens

4 slices multigrain bread (toasted and halved)

Instructions:

Combine all ingredients except salt and pepper. Give it a gentle toss. Season it with pepper and salt. Serve with toast on the side.

Zucchini and Goat Cheese Frittata

Ingredients:

1/8 tsp. pepper

2 medium zucchinis

2 oz. goat cheese (crumbled)

8 eggs

1 clove crushed garlic

2 tbsp. milk

1 tbsp. olive oil

¼ tsp. salt

Instructions:

Preheat oven to 350 degrees. Slice the zucchinis into round slices. Whisk the eggs with pepper, salt, and milk. Heat olive oil over medium heat. Add garlic and cook for 30 seconds. Add zucchini. Cook for 5 minutes. Pour whisked eggs and stir for a minute.

Top with cheese and transfer to oven. Bake for 10 minutes. Let it sit for 3 minutes. Slice into pie wedges. Serve.

Mediterranean Pasta Salad

Ingredients:

½ cup frozen peas

zest and juice of 1 lemon

8 oz. mozzarella cheese (chopped)

¼ cup chopped fresh parsley

2 tsp. olive oil

¼ cup bell pepper (chopped)

1 can artichoke hearts (chopped)

8 oz. farfalle

Instructions:

Cook pasta according to package instructions. Mix lemon zest and juice, with olive oil. Add parsley, cheese, artichoke hearts, and bell pepper. Place peas in colander. Drain pasta over peas.

Shake to drain. Toss pasta and peas to artichoke mixture. Serve warm.

Rhubarb Lentil Soup

Ingredients:

3 large rainbow chard leaves
3 tbsp. chopped fresh cilantro
2 tbsp. coconut oil
3/4 lb. rhubarb (trimmed, sliced)
¼ tsp. ground cardamom
3/4 cup French green lentils
1 medium onion (diced)
2 tsp. brown mustard seeds
6 tbsp. whole milk Greek yogurt
1 tsp. cumin seeds
2 tsp. minced garlic

1 tbsp. packed dark brown sugar

¼ tsp. ground turmeric

1 tsp. coriander seeds

kosher salt

1 tbsp. minced fresh ginger

1 small jalapeño (minced)

Instructions:

Separate the stems from chard leaves. Chop leaves and slice stems. Heat the oil over medium-high heat. Stir in cumin, mustard, and coriander seeds. Cook until mustard seeds begin to pop. Turn heat down to medium. Stir in cardamom, garlic, ginger, and turmeric. Cook for 2 minutes.

Add onion, chard stems, and jalapeño. Stir occasionally for 5 minutes. Add brown sugar, rhubarb, salt, lentils, and 5 cups water. Bring to a boil. Simmer for 30 minutes. Add chard leaves. Simmer for 5 minutes more. Season it with salt and brown sugar. Serve topped with cilantro and a dollop of Greek yogurt.

Mediterranean Chicken Stew

Ingredients:

1 cup whole-wheat couscous
3 chicken breast halves (chopped)
1 can pureed tomatoes
coarse salt and ground pepper
1 ½ pounds escarole (chopped)
1 medium onion (sliced)
½ teaspoon dried oregano
4 garlic cloves (sliced)
1 tbsp. olive oil

Instructions:

Heat the oil over medium-high heat. Season the chicken with salt and pepper. Cook until browned. Toss occasionally. Set aside.

Add oregano, onion, and garlic in pot. Season them with salt and pepper. Cook 2 to 4 minutes. Add tomatoes. Cook for 8 minutes. Add chicken. Simmer. Cover and cook 2 to 4 minutes. Add escarole. Cook until escarole is tender. Serve over couscous.

Kale & White Bean Soup with Sausage

Ingredients:

1 medium carrot (diced)
1 can cannellini beans

1 rib celery (dice)

1/8 tsp. crushed red pepper flakes

Kosher salt and freshly ground black pepper

5 large cloves garlic (minced)

½ lb. sweet Italian sausage

½ tsp. finely grated lemon zest

2 tbsp. olive oil

6 cups chicken broth

1 lb. kale (chopped)

½ small yellow onion (sliced)

1 tbsp. fresh lemon juice

Instructions:

Cut sausage into bite-size pieces. Heat olive oil in pot. Add sausage. Cook until lightly browned. Transfer sausage to a plate.

Add olive oil to pot. Increase heat to medium high. Add onion. Cook for 2 minutes. Add carrot and celery. Cook for 2 minutes. Stir in pepper flakes, garlic, salt, and pepper. Cook for 1 minute. Add chicken broth. Bring to a boil.

Reduce to medium heat. Add sausage. Mash remaining beans. Add to pot and stir. Add kale. Simmer until kale is tender. Stir in lemon juice and lemon zest. Season with salt and pepper.

Cheesy Chive Potatoes

Ingredients:

1 tbsp. butter

6 medium potatoes (cubed)

2 tbsp. minced chives

½ cup fat-free milk

1/8 tsp. pepper

½ cup feta cheese

½ tsp. salt

Instructions:

Cover potatoes with water in a saucepan. Bring to a boil. Reduce medium heat. Cover. Cook 15 minutes. Drain. Add crumbled cheese, salt, butter, milk, and pepper. Mash mixture. Stir in chives.

Sautéed Asparagus

Ingredients:

1 lb. asparagus

3 tbsp. chicken broth

3 tbsp. olive oil

2 tsp. lemon juice

2 cloves garlic

salt and pepper to taste

Instructions:

Chop garlic. Heat the broth over medium heat. Snap off bottom of asparagus stems. Cut spears into 2-inch lengths. Add the asparagus to broth. Cover and cook for 5 minutes. Transfer to a bowl. Toss asparagus with remaining ingredients while it is still hot.

Chickpea Salad

Ingredients:

1 can chickpeas (drained and rinsed)

2 tsp. olive oil

salt and pepper

6 oz. olives

1 tbsp. fresh parsley (chopped)

juice from one lemon

1 tsp. cumin

Instructions:

Place all ingredients in a bowl. Toss and stir. Serve with rice.

Couscous and Dried Cherries Salad

Ingredients:

¼ cup pine nuts, toasted

1 cup chicken broth

Salt and pepper to taste

½ cup dried cherries

1 tablespoon Dijon mustard

¼ cup sliced green onions

3 tablespoons balsamic vinegar

1 tablespoon olive oil

¾ cup uncooked couscous

½ cup chopped cucumber

½ cup chopped carrot

Instructions:

Boil broth in a saucepan. Stir in couscous. Cover and remove from heat. Let stand for 5 minutes. Fluff with a fork.

Combine onions, cherries, pine nuts, cucumber, carrot, and couscous. Combine remaining ingredients. Shake well. Pour over salad and toss. Serve.

Mediterranean Watermelon Salad

Ingredients:

1 bowl watermelon cubes
salt and pepper
2 yellow bell peppers
pistachios
rocket lettuce
jeera powder
pomegranate Juice
2 tbsp. olive oil
1 cup cucumber
oregano
10 olives
parsley (chopped)
romaine lettuce
1 tbsp. mustard paste
1 cup tomatoes
flax seeds
1 cup onions

Instructions:

Put pomegranate juice into bowl. Add salt, jeera powder, pepper, oregano, olive oil, and mustard paste. Place watermelon cubes, olives, cucumber, tomatoes, onions, and yellow bell peppers in another bowl. Add salt, parsley, and pepper. Mix well. Add flax seeds, lettuce leaves, and pistachios. Add to the watermelon mixture. Toss well. Serve chilled.

Chapter 4 – Dinner Options

Curry Rubbed Salmon with Napa Slaw

Ingredients:

1 pound Napa cabbage (sliced)

1 cup brown basmati rice

2 tsp. curry powder

4 salmon fillets

2 tbsp. grapeseed oil

½ cup fresh mint leaves

¼ cup fresh lime juice

1 pound carrots (grated)

ground pepper

some lime wedges

salt

Instructions:

Boil 2 cups water. Add rice. Season it with salt and pepper. Cover, and reduce heat to medium-low. Cook until tender.

Combine carrots, mint, oil, cabbage, and lime juice in a bowl. Season it with salt and pepper. Toss.

Place salmon in foil-lined baking sheet 10 minutes before rice is done. Rub salmon with curry. Season with salt and pepper. Broil for 8 minutes. Fluff rice with fork. Serve alongside salad and salmon.

Crisp Lamb Lettuce Wraps

Ingredients:

6 oz. lean ground lamb

2 tsp. minced fresh garlic

2 tbsp. torn mint leaves

1 tsp. ground cinnamon

¼ tsp. black pepper

8 Boston lettuce leaves

½ cup chopped parsley

¾ tsp. kosher salt

2 tsp. canola oil

1 tbsp. pine nuts

1 cup chopped onion

½ cup chopped tomato

¼ cup red pepper hummus

¼ cup Greek yogurt

½ cup chopped cucumber

Instructions:

Heat skillet over high heat. Add oil. Sauté onion. Add lamb. Sauté for 5 minutes. Add other solid ingredients. Combine tomato, cucumber, and parsley in medium bowl. Stir in lamb mixture. Combine yogurt and hummus. Place ¼ cup lamb mixture for every lettuce leaf. Top with 1 tbsp. hummus mixture. Divide mint and pine nuts evenly among wraps. Serve

Greek Lamb Chops

Ingredients:

8 lamb chops (trimmed)

1 tbsp. dried oregano

cooking spray

½ tsp. salt

¼ tsp. black pepper

1 tbsp. bottled minced garlic

2 tbsp. lemon juice

Instructions:

Preheat broiler. Combine all ingredients. Rub over both sides of chops. Place lamb chops on broiler pan coated with cooking spray. Broil 4 minutes on each side.

Chicken Kebabs

Ingredients:

250 gm. boneless chicken (minced)

1 tsp. coriander leaves (chopped)

Handful of hari mirch

1 tsp. ginger paste

1 tsp. garlic paste

1 tsp. salt

Oil

Instructions:

Mix all ingredients. Shape into small kebabs. Refrigerate for an hour. Heat oil and fry the kebabs until done.

Seared Mediterranean Tuna Steaks

Ingredients:

4 Yellow fin tuna steaks

12 chopped pitted kalamata olives

1 ½ cups chopped seeded tomato

¼ cup chopped green onions

1 tbsp. olive oil

3 tbsp. chopped fresh parsley

½ tsp. bottled minced garlic

½ tsp. salt

1/8 tsp. black pepper

½ tsp. ground coriander

1 tbsp. lemon juice

1 tbsp. capers

cooking spray

Instructions:

Heat skillet over medium-high heat. Sprinkle fish with teaspoon salt, pepper, and coriander. Coat pan with cooking spray. Add fish to pan and cook 4 minutes. Combine salt, tomato, and remaining ingredients. Serve tomato mixture on top of fish.

Greek Dinner Salad

Ingredients:

¼ cup coarsely fresh parsley (chopped)

3 tbsp. coarsely chopped fresh dill

6 cups shredded Romaine lettuce

¾ cup feta cheese

1 tbsp. olive oil

1 cucumber (thinly sliced)

1 tbsp. fresh lemon juice

1 cup red onion (sliced)

6 whole wheat pitas

1 tsp. dried oregano

3 cups diced tomato

1 tbsp. capers

1 can chickpeas

Instructions:

Combine parsley, dill, olive oil, lemon juice, and oregano. Add the rest of the ingredients. Serve with pita wedges.

Super-fast Kofte

Ingredients:

½ cup chopped white onion
1 large egg white (beaten)
¼ tsp. ground red pepper
1/3 cup dry breadcrumbs
¼ tsp. ground cinnamon
1/8 tsp. ground allspice

1 lb. lean ground round

8 slices plum tomato

¼ cup plain yogurt

¼ cup chopped mint

2 tbsp. tomato paste

1 tsp. minced garlic

½ tsp. ground cumin

Cooking spray

½ tsp. salt

4 pitas

Instructions:

Preheat broiler. Combine ingredients in a large bowl. Stir until just combined. Divide into equal portions. Shape into patties. Place patties on a pan coated with cooking spray. Broil 4 minutes. Place a slice of tomato and 1 patty in a pita half. Top with yogurt.

Greek Feta Burgers

Ingredients:

1 package frozen chopped spinach
½ cup feta cheese
¾ pound lean ground lamb
¼ cup chopped fresh mint
½ cup diced tomato
1 tbsp. lemon juice
1 egg white (beaten)
4 hamburger buns
¼ tsp. pepper
cooking spray

Instructions:

Combine spinach, lemon juice, pepper, and egg white. Stir well. Add lamb, mint, and crumbled cheese. Divide into portions and shape into patties. Coat grill with cooking spray. Grill patties for 5 minutes. Place patties on buns. Top with tomato, cucumber-dill sauce, and half a bun.

Lemon Basil Shrimp and Pasta

Ingredients:

1 lb. peeled large shrimp

2 tbsp. olive oil

8 oz. uncooked spaghetti

2 tbsp. fresh lemon juice

2 cups baby spinach

3 tbsp. drained capers

¼ cup chopped basil

3 quarts water

½ tsp. salt

Instructions:

Boil water. Add pasta. Cook 8 minutes. Add shrimp to pan. Cook 3 minutes. Drain. Place pasta in a bowl. Stir in basil and other ingredients except spinach. Place ½ cup spinach on a plate. Top with 1 cup pasta mixture. Serve on other plates.

Moussaka

Ingredients:

1 regular size eggplant (peeled and sliced into rounds)

2 cups plain whole yogurt

2 cloves garlic (minced)

¾ cup crushed tomatoes

1 cup parmesan (grated)

1 large onion (minced)

1 lb. potatoes (sliced)

3 eggs (beaten)

1 lb. ground beef

¾ cup light cream

½ teaspoon nutmeg

½ teaspoon cinnamon

butter

olive oil

Instructions:

Preheat oven to 375 degrees Fahrenheit. Brush eggplant with olive oil. Season it with salt and pepper. Brown the eggplant over medium high heat. Place on paper towel to drain. Cook onion and garlic for 3 minutes. Add ground beef. Add spices. Add tomatoes. Simmer for 10 minutes.

Brown potato slices on another skillet. Place on paper towel to drain. Season them with salt and pepper. Layer the potatoes in a buttered baking dish. Add eggplant and meat. Top with parmesan. Combine cream, eggs and yogurt in a bowl. Season them with salt and pepper. Pour over casserole. Let it sit for 10 minutes. Bake for 40 minutes. Allow casserole to sit for 15 minutes.

Dirty Potatoes

Ingredients:

1/3 cup pitted kalamata olives

2 tbsp. olive oil

2 lbs. small new potatoes (halved)

Instructions:

Preheat oven to 400 degrees Fahrenheit. Spread potatoes on a baking sheet. Drizzle with oil. Toss. Bake for 45 minutes. Puree olives. Scrape puree over potatoes and toss. Transfer to bowl. Serve hot.

Chopped Greek Chicken Salad

Ingredients:

½ cup red onion (chopped)

1 medium cucumber (chopped)

2 tbsp. olive oil

6 cups chopped romaine lettuce

2 ½ cups chopped cooked chicken

1 tbsp. chopped fresh dill

½ cup feta cheese

1 tsp. garlic powder

¼ tsp. salt

2 medium tomatoes (chopped)

¼ tsp. freshly ground pepper

1/3 cup red-wine vinegar

½ cup sliced ripe black olives

Instructions:

Whisk salt, oil, garlic powder, dill, vinegar, and pepper. Add chicken, cucumber, tomatoes, lettuce, crumbled feta, olives, and onion. Toss to coat. Serve.

Chapter 5 – Snacks and Other Sides

Marinated Olives plus Feta

Ingredients:

1 tsp. rosemary (chopped)
pinch of crushed red pepper
2 tbsp. olive oil
1 cup sliced pitted olives
freshly ground pepper
zest and juice of 1 lemon
½ cup diced feta cheese
2 cloves garlic (sliced)

Instructions:

Combine all ingredients in a medium bowl. Toss to coat. You may refrigerate for one day before serving.

Mediterranean Pick Me Up Snack

Ingredients:

1 slice whole-wheat bread (bite-size pieces)

10 cherry tomatoes

¼ oz. sliced aged cheese

6 oil-cured olives

Instructions:

Combine bread pieces, tomatoes, cheese and olives in a portable container.

Quick Mediterranean Dip

Ingredients:

minced herbs (basil, parsley, dill, and mint)
1/3 cup plain nonfat yogurt
1 package feta cheese
1/3 cup nonfat sour cream
fresh ground black pepper
1 tsp. garlic (minced)
¼ teaspoon sea salt

Instructions:

In a blender or a food processor, puree all ingredients until smooth; serve as a spread or dip with warm pita bread.

Creamy Artichoke Dip

Ingredients:

4 slices white bread (cut into 2-inch pieces)

3 tbsp. fresh squeezed lemon juice

chopped chives

1 box artichoke hearts

2 anchovy fillets

ground pepper

½ tsp. sugar

2/3 cup olive oil

coarse salt

Instructions:

Pour one cup of water over bread. Squeeze water out bread then put in a food processor. Add sugar, artichokes, and anchovies. Blend into a smooth paste. While processing, pour oil through feed tube. Add lemon juice. Keep whirling until mixture becomes creamy. Season it with salt and pepper. Place in a dish. Drizzle with oil. Sprinkle with fresh chives. Serve with bread.

Potato Croquettes with Parmesan

Ingredients:

2 cups mashed potatoes

2 tbsp. vegetable oil

2 tbsp. minced onions

3 tbsp. grated parmesan

¾ cup breadcrumbs

2 tbsp. parsley (minced)

1 egg (beaten)

Instructions:

Blend the following thoroughly: onion, parsley, egg, potato, and cheese. Shape into patties. Refrigerate. Fry croquettes in hot oil until brown. Serve hot.

Mediterranean Hummus

Ingredients:

1 clove chopped garlic

1 clove garlic

2 tbsp. olive oil

4 tbsp. lemon juice

1 can garbanzo beans

2 tbsp. tahini

1 tsp. salt

black pepper

Instructions:

Put garlic and garbanzo beans into blender. Blend ingredients. Reserve a tablespoon of garbanzo for garnish. Add tahini, salt, lemon juice, chopped garlic. Blend everything until creamy. Serve in a bowl. Sprinkle with pepper and drizzled with olive oil. Garnish with reserved garbanzo.

Pine Nuts and Spinach Orzo

Ingredients:

½ tsp. crushed red pepper flakes
2 cups feta cheese
1 cup pine nuts

¼ tsp. pepper

1 minced garlic clove

½ tsp. dried basil

1 pack orzo pasta

1 tbsp. butter

2 packs baby spinach

¼ cup olive oil

¼ cup balsamic vinegar

1 large tomato (chopped)

1 tsp. salt

Instructions:

Cook pasta as per package instructions. Cook pine nuts, pepper flakes basil, and garlic, in oil and butter just until lightly browned. Add pepper, salt, and spinach. Stir for 5 minutes. Drain pasta. Add to spinach mixture. Drizzle with vinegar. Sprinkle with crumbled cheese and tomato.

Simple Mediterranean Layered Dip

Ingredients:

1 cup chopped tomatoes, cucumbers, and chopped black olives

½ cup Miracle Whip spread

pita bread wedges

cracked peppercorns

250 g cream cheese

1 pack feta

oregano

tomatoes

cheese

Instructions:

Mix Miracle Whip with cream cheese. Spread on serving platter. Top with cucumbers, olives, and tomatoes. Sprinkle with cheese. Serve with pita bread wedges.

Basic Greek Salad

Ingredients:

3 large tomatoes (chopped)

6 black Greek olives (sliced)

1 cup feta cheese

2 cucumbers (chopped)

¼ cup olive oil

4 tsp. lemon juice

1 ½ tsp. dried oregano

1 small red onion (chopped)

salt and pepper

Instructions:

Mix tomatoes, onion, and cucumber. Sprinkle with oil. Add lemon juice. Mix in oregano, salt, and pepper. Sprinkle feta cheese and olives. Serve.

Creamy Mediterranean Dip

Ingredients:

1/3 cup chopped black olives

250 gram cream cheese (softened)

1/4 cup onions (chopped)

1/3 cup sun-dried tomatoes

2 tbsp. light sour cream

Instructions:

Mix sour cream and cream cheese. Add other ingredients and mix well. Serve with fresh vegetables.

Tzatziki

Ingredients:

3 ½ tbsp. olive oil
2 cups Greek yogurt
2 cloves minced garlic
1 ½ tbsp. red wine vinegar
1 cucumber (grated)
salt

Instructions:

Whisk together yogurt, garlic, and cucumber. Stir in olive oil. Add red wine vinegar. Mix well. Season it with salt.

5 Layer Greek Dip

Ingredients:

¼ cup chopped cucumbers

1 pack (4 oz.) feta cheese (crumbled)

2 tbsp. sliced kalamata olives

1 pack hummus

½ cup chopped tomatoes

pita chips

Instructions:

Spread hummus on a pie plate. Cover with layers of other ingredients. Serve with chips.

8 Layer Mediterranean Dip

Ingredients:

¼ cup feta cheese

1 cup baby spinach (chopped)

1 cup sliced roasted red peppers

6 oz. jar marinated artichoke hearts (chopped)

¼ cup onions (sliced)

1 cup nonfat Greek-style yogurt

½ cup sliced pitted black olives

8 oz. hummus

pita chips

Instructions:

Spread hummus evenly on a square dish. Add layer of spinach. Add a layer of peppers. Add a layer of artichokes hearts. Spread an even layer of yogurt. Sprinkle with green onions, crumbled feta, and olives. Serve with pita chips

Quick Mediterranean Egg Snack

Ingredients:

4 hard-boiled eggs (sliced)
½ tsp. kosher salt
½ tsp. paprika
1 tsp. olive oil

Instructions:

Dip egg slices in oil. Sprinkle with salt and paprika. Serve on plate.

Conclusion

Thank you again for downloading this book!

I hope this book was able to help you to discover the wonders of the Mediterranean flavors.

The next step of course is to include the recipes described here in your menu plan to help you reduce your calorie intake and eventually help you lose weight.

Part 2

Breakfast Recipes

Creamy Date Smoothie

Start your morning with a blended drink that is really nutritious and delicious… This shake is a great way to use healthy dates in your diet. Almond butter adds a delish richness in smoothie.

Serves: 2 persons
Preparation Time: 10 minutes

Ingredients:

- 4 Medjool date, pitted and chopped roughly
- 1 cup fat-free plain Greek yogurt
- 2 tablespoons almond butter
- 1 cup fresh apple juice
- 1 cup ice cubes, crushed

Directions:

1. In a high speed blender, add all ingredients and pulse till smooth and creamy.

2. Transfer into 2 serving glasses and serve immediately.

Nutritional Information per Serving:

Calories: 293
Fat: 9.5g
Carbohydrates: 35.9g
Dietary Fiber: 2g
Protein: 18.7g

Toast with Avocado

One of the simple but delicious breakfast... Mashed avocado over toasted bread is surprisingly filling too. This recipe of avocado toast makes a wonderful breakfast for whole family.

Serves: 4 persons
Preparation Time: 15 minutes
Cooking Time: 16 minutes

Ingredients:

- 1 large avocado, peeled, pitted and chopped roughly
- ¼ teaspoon fresh lemon juice

- 2 tablespoons fresh mint leaves, chopped finely
- Salt and freshly ground black pepper, to taste
- 4 large rye bread slices
- 2 tablespoons feta cheese, crumbled

Directions:

1. In a bowl, add avocado and with a fork, mash roughly.
2. Add lemon juice, mint, salt and black pepper and stir to combine well and keep aside.
3. Heat a nonstick frying pan on medium-high heat and toast the slice for about 2 minutes per side.
4. Repeat with the remaining slices.
5. Spread the avocado mixture over each slice evenly.
6. Sprinkle with feta and serve immediately.

Nutritional Information per Serving:

Calories: 301
Fat: 10.4g
Carbohydrates: 41.6g
Dietary Fiber: 7.9g
Protein: 7.1g

Fruity Yogurt Parfait

A delicious and quick breakfast recipe that is really easy to assemble... This parfait is loaded with the delish flavors of Greek yogurt, fruit and almonds. Toasted almonds add a wonderfully nutty crunch in parfait.

Serves: 4 persons
Preparation Time: 15 minutes
Cooking Time: 8-10 minutes

Ingredients:

- 2 cups fat-free plain Greek yogurt
- ¼ cup honey, divided
- ¼ cup water
- 2 tablespoons sugar
- ½ teaspoon fresh lime zest, grated finely

- ¼ teaspoon ground cinnamon
- ¼ teaspoon vanilla extract
- 2 peaches, pitted and quartered
- 4 plums, pitted and quartered
- ¼ cup almonds, toasted and chopped

Directions:

1. In a bowl, add yogurt and honey and mix till well combined and keep aside.
2. In a pan, mix together water, sugar, lime zest, cinnamon, vanilla extract and remaining ingredients on medium heat.
3. Stir in peaches and plums and cook, stirring occasionally for about 8-10 minutes or till fruits becomes tender.
4. Remove from heat and keep aside to cool completely.
5. Divide half of the yogurt mixture in 4 tall serving glasses evenly.
6. Divide the fruit mixture over yogurt evenly.
7. Place remaining yogurt over fruit mixture.

8. Garnish with almonds and serve.

Nutritional Information per Serving:

Calories: 255
Fat: 5.1g
Carbohydrates: 39.1g
Dietary Fiber: 2g
Protein: 14.7g

Couscous with Dried Fruit

A quick and tasty breakfast treat for whole family… Combo of dried fruit, milk and butter with couscous makes such a hearty breakfast. Surely this dish will become family favorite.

Serves: 4 persons
Preparation Time: 10 minutes
Cooking Time: 8-10 minutes

Ingredients:

- 3 cups low-fat milk
- 1 cup uncooked whole-wheat couscous
- ¼ cup dried currants
- 1/3 cup dried apricots, chopped

- 6 teaspoons dark brown sugar, divided
- ¼ teaspoon ground cinnamon
- Salt, to taste
- 2 teaspoons unsalted butter, melted

Directions:

1. In a pan, heat milk for about 2-3 minutes on medium-high heat.
2. Remove from heat and immediately, stir in couscous, dried fruit, 4 teaspoons of brown sugar, cinnamon and salt.
3. Keep aside, covered for about 15 minutes.
4. In 4 serving bowls, divide the couscous mixture.
5. Top with melted butter and remaining brown sugar evenly and serve immediately.

Nutritional Information per Serving:

Calories: 284
Fat: 4.1g
Carbohydrates: 49.5g

Dietary Fiber: 2.8g
Protein: 12g

Mixed Veggie Omelet

One of the fantastic way to start your day... This recipe makes a perfect fluffy omelet for your breakfast. Sautéed vegetables with feta cheese and eggs makes a perfect combination in this omelet.

Serves: 4 persons
Preparation Time: 15 minutes
Cooking Time: 15 minutes

Ingredients:

- 1 teaspoon olive oil
- 2 cups fresh fennel bulb, sliced thinly
- ¼ cup canned artichoke hearts, rinsed, drained and chopped
- ¼ cup green olives, pitted and chopped
- 1 Roma tomato, chopped
- 6 eggs

- Salt and freshly ground black pepper, to taste
- ½ cup goat cheese, crumbled

Directions:

1. Preheat the oven to 325 degrees F.
2. In a large ovenproof skillet, heat the oil on medium-high heat.
3. Add the chopped fennel bulb and sauté for about 5 minutes.
4. Stir in artichoke, olives and tomato and cook for about 3 minutes.
5. Meanwhile in a bowl, add eggs, salt and black pepper and beat till well combined.
6. Place the egg mixture over veggie mixture and stir to combine.
7. Cook for about 2 minutes.
8. Sprinkle with the goat cheese evenly and immediately, transfer the skillet into the oven.
9. Bake for about 5 minutes or till eggs are set completely.

10. Remove the skillet from oven and carefully transfer the omelet onto a cutting board.

11. Cut into desired size wedges and serve.

Nutritional Information per Serving:

Calories: 208
Fat: 13.8g
Carbohydrates: 8g
Dietary Fiber: 2.7g
Protein: 14.1g

Scrambled Eggs with Veggies

A super quick and easy meal for busy life... This delicious recipe of scrambled eggs with feta cheese, spinach and tomato... This recipe makes a perfect blend of fresh veggies, feta cheese and eggs.

Serves: 2 persons
Preparation Time: 10 minutes
Cooking Time: 8minutes

Ingredients:

- 1 tablespoon olive oil
- 1 cup fresh baby spinach
- 1/3 cup tomato, chopped
- 3 eggs, beaten
- 2 tablespoons feta cheese, cubed
- Salt and freshly ground black pepper, to taste

Directions:

1. In a large frying pan, heat oil on medium heat.
2. Add spinach and tomatoes and sauté for about 3-4 minutes.
3. Add eggs and cook, stirring continuously for about 1 minute.
4. Stir in feta and cook for about 2 minutes or till set according to desired doneness.
5. Stir in salt and black pepper and remove from heat.
6. Serve immediately.

Nutritional Information per Serving:

Calories: 201
Fat: 16.5g
Carbohydrates: 2.8g
Dietary Fiber: 0.7g
Protein: 11g

Cheesy Veggie Muffins

A variety of fresh vegetables combined with eggs, Asiago cheese and feta cheese provides a perfect start to the day... These colorful vegetables go perfectly with cheeses and eggs.

Serves: 8 persons
Preparation Time: 15 minutes
Cooking Time: 10-12 minutes

Ingredients:

- ¼ cup half-and-half
- 6 large eggs
- Salt and freshly ground black pepper, to taste
- ½ cup sun-dried tomatoes in oil, drained and chopped

- 1/3 cup canned kalamata olives, drained, pitted and quartered
- ¼ cup bottled sweet red peppers, drained and chopped
- ¼ cup canned artichokes in oil, drained and sliced thinly
- ¼ cup Asiago cheese, shredded
- ¼ cup feta cheese, crumbled
- ¼ cup fresh parsley, chopped

Directions:

1. Preheat the oven to 375 degrees F. Grease 24 cups of mini muffin tins.
2. In a bowl, add cup half-and-half, eggs, salt and black pepper and black pepper and beat well.
3. In another large bowl, mix together vegetables and Asiago cheese.
4. Place the egg mixture into prepared muffin cups about ¾ of full.
5. Place vegetables mixture over egg mixture evenly and top with remaining egg mixture.

6. Sprinkle with feta and parsley evenly.
7. Bake for about 10-12 minutes or till eggs are done completely.

Nutritional Information per Serving:

Calories: 92
Fat: 6.5g
Carbohydrates: 2.4g
Dietary Fiber: 0.7g
Protein: 6.3g

Cheesy Zucchini Frittata

A protein packed breakfast for whole family... This so easy to prepare frittata is a great way to use garden fresh zucchini in a flavorful breakfast meal. Definitely whole family will love to enjoy this frittata.

Serves: 4 persons
Preparation Time: 15 minutes
Cooking Time: 19 minutes

Ingredients:

- 2 tablespoons milk
- 8 eggs

- Salt and freshly ground black pepper, to taste
- 1 tablespoon olive oil
- 1 garlic clove, minced
- 2 medium zucchinis, cut into ¼-inch thick round slices
- ½ cup goat cheese, crumbled

Directions:

1. Preheat the oven to 350 degrees F.
2. In a bowl, add cup milk, eggs, salt and black pepper and black pepper and beat well. Keep aside.
3. In an ovenproof skillet, heat oil on medium heat.
4. Add garlic and sauté for about 1 minute.
5. Stir in zucchini and cook for about 5 minutes.
6. Add the egg mixture and stir for about 1 minute.
7. Sprinkle the cheese on top evenly.

8. Immediately, transfer the skillet in the oven.
9. Bake for about 10-12 minutes or till eggs become set.
10. Remove from oven and keep aside to cool for about 3-5 minutes.
11. Cut into desired size wedges and serve.

Nutritional Information per Serving:

Calories: 241
Fat: 17.6g
Carbohydrates: 4.9g
Dietary Fiber: 1.1g
Protein: 16.9g

Oats Pancakes

One of the hearty and healthy pancakes for whole family… These healthy pancakes are packed with protein. Yogurt is a key ingredient that makes these pancakes really fluffy and tasty enough.

Serves: 6 persons
Preparation Time: 10 minutes
Cooking Time: 4 minutes

Ingredients:

- ½ cup all-purpose flour
- 1 cup old-fashioned oats
- 2 tablespoons flax seeds
- 1 teaspoon baking soda
- Salt, to taste
- 2 tablespoons agave syrup
- 2 large eggs
- 2 cups plain Greek yogurt
- 2 tablespoons canola oil

Directions:

1. In a blender, add flour, oats, flax seeds, baking soda and salt and pulse till well combined.
2. Transfer the mixture into a large bowl.
3. Add remaining ingredients except oil and mix till well combined.

4. Keep aside for about 20 minutes before cooking.
5. Heat a large nonstick skillet on medium heat and grease with a little oil.
6. Add ¼ cup of the mixture and cook for about 2 minutes or till bottom becomes golden brown.
7. Carefully, flip the side and cook for about 2 minutes more.
8. Repeat with the remaining mixture.

Nutritional Information per Serving:

Calories: 232
Fat: 9.5g
Carbohydrates: 22.6g
Dietary Fiber: 1.6g
Protein: 3.8g

Yogurt Crepes

A family friendly breakfast recipe… These elegant baked crepes are filled with smooth, creamy and nutrient rich Greek yogurt. Yogurt gives softness and creaminess to these crepes.

Serves: 8 persons
Preparation Time: 10 minutes
Cooking Time: 15 minutes

Ingredients:

- 2cups flour
- 1/3 cup sugar plus extra for dusting
- 1 teaspoon baking powder
- ¼ teaspoon baking soda
- Salt, to taste
- 4-ounce frozen butter
- ½ cup plain Greek yogurt
- 1 large egg

Directions:

1. Preheat the oven to 400 degrees F.
2. In a bowl, mix together flour, sugar, baking powder, baking soda and salt.
3. Reserve some flour mixture in another bowl.
4. Grate the butter in flour mixture and stir to combine.

5. Add yogurt and egg and mix till well combined and a chunky dough forms.
6. Onto a floured surface, place the dough and knead till a sticky dough forms.
7. With a rolling pin, roll the dough onto a floured surface to an 8-inch circle.
8. Dust with the reserved flour mixture and with your hands press down the slightly.
9. Sprinkle with the extra sugar.
10. Cut into equal sized 8 wedges and arrange onto a large baking sheet.
11. Bake for about 15 minutes.

Nutritional Information per Serving:

Calories: 356
Fat: 16.6g
Carbohydrates: 1.1g
Dietary Fiber: 44.4g
Protein: 8g

Lunch Recipes

Cucumber & Olives Salad

An excellent salad that is really refreshing, light but yummy enough... This refreshing salad is a great choice for light lunch. Fresh lemon juice gives the vegetables a delish tanginess.

Serves: 6 persons
Preparation Time: 15 minutes

Ingredients:

- 2 cucumbers, peeled and chopped
- 3 large ripe tomatoes, chopped
- ½ cup black olives, pitted and sliced
- 1 small red onion, chopped
- 4 teaspoons fresh lemon juice
- ¼ cup olive oil
- 1½ teaspoon dried oregano, crushed
- Salt and freshly ground black pepper, to taste
- 1 cup feta cheese, crumbled

Directions:

1. In a large serving bowl, add all ingredients except feta and toss to coat well.
2. Top with feta and serve immediately.

Nutritional Information per Serving:

Calories: 189
Fat: 15.3g
Carbohydrates: 10.3g
Dietary Fiber: 2.4g
Protein: 5.3g

Chickpeas & veggie Gazpacho

A simple and easy summer gazpacho that is really delicious ... Combo of chickpeas and vegetables with tomato juice makes this delicious soup filling too. Curry powder and hot pepper sauce gives a spicy kick to this gazpacho.

Serves: 10 persons
Preparation Time: 20 minutes

Ingredients:

- 1 (15½-ounce) can chickpeas, drained and rinsed
- 1 large plum tomato, chopped
- 1 cucumber, peeled, seeded and chopped finely
- 1 celery stalk, chopped finely
- ½ of yellow bell pepper, seeded and chopped finely
- ½ of red bell pepper, seeded and chopped finely
- 2 tablespoons sweet onion, chopped finely
- 2 scallions, chopped
- 1 garlic clove, minced
- ¼ cup fresh parsley, chopped
- 1 (46 fl. oz.) can tomato juice
- 1 tablespoon fresh lemon juice
- Dash of hot pepper sauce
- 1 teaspoon curry powder
- Pinch of dried oregano, crushed

- Freshly ground black pepper, to taste

Directions:

1. In a large glass bowl, add all ingredients add all ingredients and gently stir to combine.//
2. Cover and refrigerate to chill for about 2 hours before serving.

Nutritional Information per Serving:

Calories: 217
Fat: 3g
Carbohydrates: 39.8g
Dietary Fiber: 9.9g
Protein: 11.1g

Lamb Filled Pita with Yogurt Sauce

A great light and delicious meal that is really enjoyable for lunch… These pita pockets are filled with juicy and mouthwatering lamb and the topped with cool and tangy yogurt sauce.

Serves: 4 persons
Preparation Time: 15 minutes
Cooking Time: 4-5 minutes

Ingredients:

- 2 teaspoons olive oil
- 2 garlic clove, minced
- 1 tablespoon fresh rosemary, minced
- Salt and freshly ground black pepper, to taste
- ¾ pound boneless leg of lamb, cut into bite sized pieces
- 1 (6-ounce) container plat fat-free plain Greek yogurt
- 1½ cups cucumber, chopped finely
- 1 tablespoon fresh lemon juice
- 4 (6-ounce) whole-wheat pita breads, warmed

Directions:

1. In a large nonstick skillet, heat oil on medium-high heat.
2. In a bowl, mix together garlic, rosemary, salt and black pepper.
3. Add lamb and toss to coat well.

4. Transfer the lamb mixture into skillet and stir fry for about 4-5 minutes or till desired doneness.

5. Meanwhile for yogurt sauce in a bowl, mix together yogurt, cucumber, lemon juice, salt and black pepper.

6. Transfer the lamb mixture between all the pitas evenly.

7. Serve immediately with the drizzling of the yogurt sauce.

Nutritional Information per Serving:

Calories: 385
Fat: 10.4g
Carbohydrates: 39.7g
Dietary Fiber: 5.4g
Protein: 34.8g

Chickpea Patties

A super-fast recipe for family and friend's luncheon gathering... Even meat lovers would love to eat these meatless patties. Chickpeas patties make a wonderful pairing with lettuce and yogurt sauce.

Serves: 4 persons
Preparation Time: 15 minutes
Cooking Time: 4-6 minutes

Ingredients:

- 1 (15½-ounce) can chickpeas, drained and rinsed
- 1 garlic clove, chopped
- ½ cup fresh parsley, chopped roughly
- ¼ teaspoon ground cumin
- Salt and freshly ground black pepper, to taste
- ¼ cup all-purpose flour, divided
- 1 egg, beaten
- 2 tablespoons olive oil
- 8 cups lettuce leaves, torn
- ½ cup low-fat plain Greek yogurt
- 2 tablespoons fresh lemon juice

Directions:

1. In a food processor, add chickpeas, garlic, parsley, cumin, salt and black pepper and pulse till chopped.

2. Transfer the mixture into a bowl.
3. Add 2 tablespoons of flour and egg and mix till well combined.
4. Make 8 equal sized patties from mixture.
5. In a shallow dish, place remaining flour.
6. Coat the patties with roll evenly and shake off excess flour.
7. In a large nonstick skillet, heat oil on medium-high heat.
8. Add patties and cook for about 2-3 minutes from both sides or till golden browned.
9. Meanwhile for yogurt sauce in a bowl, mix together yogurt, lemon juice, salt and black pepper.
10. Divide the lettuce between serving plates evenly.
11. Place 2 patties in each plate over greens.
12. Serve immediately with the drizzling of the yogurt sauce.

Nutritional Information per Serving:

Calories: 272
Fat: 9.8g
Carbohydrates: 37.7g
Dietary Fiber: 6.4g
Protein: 10g

Stuffed Tomatoes

A flavor packed recipe of tomatoes with a little ingredients… This plate of stuffed tomatoes will be a great choice for lunch. Surely you would love to make his recipe again and again.

Serves: 2 persons
Preparation Time: 15 minutes
Cooking Time: 5 minutes

Ingredients:

- 2 large tomatoes, halved crosswise
- ¼ cup Kalamata olives, pitted and sliced
- 2 tablespoons fresh basil, chopped
- ¼ cup goat cheese, crumbled
- ½ cup packaged garlic croutons

- 2 tablespoons low-fat balsamic vinaigrette

Directions:

1. Preheat the broiler. Set the oven rack from the 4-5-nches from heating element.
2. With your fingers, remove the seeds from the tomato halves.
3. Carefully, run a small knife vertically around the pulp, not touching the bottom.
4. Gently remove the pulp then chop it and transfer into a bowl.
5. Arrange the tomatoes over paper towels, cut side down to drain.
6. In the bowl of tomato pulp, sad remaining ingredients and mix.
7. Stuff the tomatoes with olive mixture evenly.
8. Arrange the tomatoes onto a broiler pan.
9. Broil for about 5 minutes or till cheese melted

Nutritional Information per Serving:

Calories: 202
Fat: 12.1g
Carbohydrates: 18.3g
Dietary Fiber: 2.8g
Protein: 7.1g

Veggie Pizza

An ultimate tasty treat for pizza lovers... This crispy pizza that is really healthy and a real fun to prepare at home. This pizza is packed with the flavors of nutritious veggies, basil and bubbly cheese.

Serves: 5 persons
Preparation Time: 15 minutes
Cooking Time: 10-12 minutes

Ingredients:

- 1 (12-inch) prepared pizza crust
- ¼ teaspoon Italian seasoning
- ¼ teaspoon red pepper flakes, crushed
- 1 cup goat cheese, crumbled

- 1 (14-ounce) can quartered artichoke hearts
- 3 plum tomatoes, sliced into ¼-inch thick size
- 6 kalamata olives, pitted and sliced
- ¼ cup fresh basil, chopped

Directions:

1. Preheat the oven to 450 degrees F. Grease a baking sheet.
2. Sprinkle the pizza crust with Italian seasoning and red pepper flakes evenly.
3. Place the goat cheese over crust evenly, leaving about ½-inch of the sides.
4. With the back of a spoon, gently press the cheese downwards.
5. Place the artichoke, tomato and olives on top.
6. Place the pizza crust onto prepared baking sheet.

7. Bake for about 10-12 minutes or till cheese becomes bubbly.
8. Remove from oven and sprinkle with basil.
9. Cut into equal sized wedges and serve.

Nutritional Information per Serving:

Calories: 305
Fat: 10.9g
Carbohydrates: 40.1g
Dietary Fiber: 6.2g
Protein: 14.9g

Chicken & Veggie Kebabs

A super fabulous meal for lunch that is really mouthwatering… Marinade of lemon juice, vinegar, cumin and herbs adds a flavorful touch in chicken. Flavorful chicken makes a great combo with veggies.

Serves: 8 persons
Preparation Time: 20 minutes
Cooking Time: 10 minutes

Ingredients:

- ¼ cup white vinegar
- ¼ cup fresh lemon juice
- ¼ cup olive oil
- 2 garlic cloves, minced
- ½ teaspoon dried thyme, crushed
- ½ teaspoon dried oregano, crushed
- 1 teaspoon ground cumin
- Salt and freshly ground black pepper, to taste
- 2 pounds skinless, boneless chicken breast, cubed into ½-inch size
- 1 large orange bell pepper, seeded and cubed into 1-inch size
- 1 large green bell pepper, seeded and cubed into 1-inch size
- 16 fresh mushrooms
- 16 cherry tomatoes
- 1 large onion, quartered and separated into pieces

Directions:

1. In a large bowl, mix together vinegar, lemon juice oil, garlic, dried herbs, cumin, salt and black pepper.
2. Add chicken and coat with mixture generously.
3. Cover and refrigerate to marinate for about 2-4 hours.
4. Preheat the outdoor grill to medium-high heat. Grease the grill grate.
5. Remove the chicken from refrigerator and discard the excess marinade.
6. Thread the chicken and vegetables onto pre-soaked wooden skewers evenly.
7. Grill for about 10 minutes, flipping occasionally or till desired doneness.

Nutritional Information per Serving:

Calories:214
Fat:11.2g
Carbohydrates:15.7g
Dietary Fiber:4.7g
Protein:29.4g

Herbed Pasta with Tomatoes

An easy and delicious pasta recipe with wonderful tomato sauce… Garlic and mixed herbs makes tomato sauce really flavorful. Surely your kids would ask for this recipe again and again.

Serves: 4 persons
Preparation Time: 10 minutes
Cooking Time: 15 minutes

Ingredients:

- 1 (8-ounce) package linguini pasta
- 2 tablespoons olive oil
- 1 tablespoon garlic, minced
- 1 tablespoon dried oregano, crushed
- 1 tablespoon dried basil, crushed
- 1 teaspoon dried thyme, crushed
- 2 cups plum tomatoes, chopped

Directions:

1. In a large pan of lightly salted boiling water cook for about 8-10 minutes or

according to package's directions. Drain well.
2. In a large skillet, heat oil on medium heat.
3. Add garlic and sauté for about 1 minute.
4. Stir in herbs and sauté for about 1 minute more.
5. Add pasta and cook for about 2-3 minutes or till heated completely.
6. Fold in tomatoes and remove from heat.
7. Serve hot.

Nutritional Information per Serving:

Calories:297
Fat:8.3g
Carbohydrates:47g
Dietary Fiber:2.6g
Protein:8.3g

Couscous with Cauliflower & Dates

A perfect and tasty choice of a light lunch… This luncheon dish is packed with sweet and tangy delish flavors. Make this dish for your family and receive a huge appreciation.

Serves: 4 persons
Preparation Time: 15 minutes
Cooking Time: 10 minutes

Ingredients:

- 2 tablespoons olive oil, divided
- 2 garlic cloves, minced
- 1¼ cups vegetable broth
- 1 cup pearl couscous
- 1 tablespoon fresh lemon juice
- 1 shallot, chopped
- 2 cups cauliflower florets
- Salt and freshly ground black pepper, to taste
- 3 tablespoons dates, pitted and chopped
- 1 teaspoon red wine vinegar
- 2 tablespoons fresh parsley, chopped

Directions:

1. For couscous in a large pan, heat 1 tablespoon of oil on medium-high heat.
2. Add garlic and sauté for about 1 minute.
3. Add broth and bring to a boil.
4. Stir in couscous and reduce the heat to medium.
5. Cover and simmer, stirring occasionally for about 8-10 minutes or till done completely.
6. Stir in lemon juice and remove from heat.
7. Meanwhile in a skillet, heat remaining oil on medium heat.
8. Add shallot and sauté for about 6 minutes.
9. Stir in dates and cook for about 2 minutes.
10. Stir in vinegar, salt and black pepper and transfer into the pan with couscous and stir to combine.
11. Serve warm with the garnishing of parsley.

Nutritional Information per Serving:

Calories: 276
Fat: 8g
Carbohydrates: 43.7g
Dietary Fiber: 2g
Protein: 8.4g

Prawns with Garlic Sauce

A wonderful addition in your lunch menu list… This simple and quick recipe of prawns in garlic sauce makes a wonderfully delicious meal. This garlic sauce balances the flavor of prawns in a great way.

Serves: 4 persons
Preparation Time: 15 minutes
Cooking Time: 6-8 minutes

Ingredients:

For Garlic Sauce:

- 3 garlic cloves, minced
- 1 cup fresh cilantro leaves, chopped finely
- 1 tablespoon dry white wine

- 2 tablespoons fresh lime juice
- 1 tablespoon olive oil
- ½ tablespoon red pepper flakes, crushed
- Salt, to taste

For prawns:

- 1½ pound prawns, peeled and deveined
- 2 tablespoons olive oil
- Salt and freshly ground black pepper, to taste

Directions:

1. Preheat the grill to medium-high heat. Grease the grill grate.
2. For sauce in a bowl, add all ingredients and mix till well combined. Keep aside.
3. For prawns in a bowl, add all ingredients and toss to coat well.
4. Thread the prawns onto pre-soaked wooden skewers.

5. Grill for about 3-4 minutes per side or till desired doneness.
6. In serving plates, divide the prawns and top with garlic sauce and serve.

Nutritional Information per Serving:

Calories: 303
Fat: 13.5g
Carbohydrates: 4.6g
Dietary Fiber: 0g
Protein: 39.1g

Dinner Recipes

Beans & Spinach Soup

One of the comforting, hearty and filling soup that is delicious as well… This soup is chock full of white kidney beans and spinach. Surely this soup makes a full meal for family dinner.

Serves: 6 persons
Preparation Time: 10 minutes
Cooking Time: 25 minutes

Ingredients:

- 1 tablespoon olive oil
- 1 celery stalk, chopped
- 1 onion, chopped
- 1 garlic clove, minced
- ¼ teaspoon dried thyme, crushed
- 2 (16-ounce) cans white kidney beans, rinsed and drained
- 2 cups vegetable broth
- 2 cups water
- 3 cups fresh spinach, chopped
- Salt and freshly ground black pepper, to taste
- 1 tablespoon fresh lemon juice

Directions:

1. In a large soup pan, heat oil on medium heat.
2. Add celery and onion and sauté for about 3-4 minutes.
3. Add garlic and thyme sauté for about 1 minute.

4. Stir in beans, broth and water and bring to a boil.
5. Reduce the heat to low and simmer for about 15 minutes.
6. Remove from heat and with a slotted spoon, transfer about 2 cups of the beans mixture in a bowl.
7. Keep aside to cool slightly.
8. In a blender add 2 cups of the bean mixture and pulse till smooth.
9. Return the pureed mixture in the soup and stir to combine.
10. Place the pan on medium heat and stir in spinach, salt and black pepper and cook for about 3-4 minutes.
11. Stir in lemon juice and serve hot.

Nutritional Information per Serving:

Calories: 549
Fat: 4.1g
Carbohydrates: 93.6g
Dietary Fiber: 38.4g
Protein: 38g

Seafood Stew

An impressive and crowd pleasing meal for dinner… The combination of wine, clam juice, tomato paste tomatoes, garlic makes a unique and magnificent pairing with seafood.

Serves: 6 persons
Preparation Time: 15 minutes
Cooking Time: 25 minutes

Ingredients:

- 1 tablespoon olive oil
- 1 medium onion, chopped finely
- 2 garlic clove, minced
- ¼ teaspoon red pepper flakes, crushed
- ½ pound plum tomatoes, seeded and chopped
- 1/3 cup white wine
- 1 cup clam juice
- 1 tablespoon tomato paste
- Salt, to taste

- 1 pound large shrimp, peeled and deveined
- 1 pound snapper fillets, cubed into 1-inch size
- ½ pound sea scallops
- 1/3 cup fresh parsley, minced
- 1 teaspoon fresh lemon zest, grated finely

Directions:

1. In a large Dutch oven , heat oil on medium heat.
2. Add onion and sauté for about 3-4 minutes.
3. Add garlic and red pepper flakes and sauté for about 1 minute.
4. Add tomatoes and cook for about 2 minutes.
5. Add wine, clam juice, tomato paste and salt and bring to a boil.
6. Reduce the heat to low and simmer, covered for about 10 minutes.

7. Stir in seafood and simmer, covered for about 6-8 minutes.
8. Stir in parsley and remove from heat.
9. Serve hot with the garnishing of lemon zest.

Nutritional Information per Serving:

Calories: 263
Fat: 4.2g
Carbohydrates: 11.8g
Dietary Fiber: 1.3g
Protein: 41.3g

Salmon with Veggies

A combination of delicious and nutrient filled ingredients… This combination makes a really delicious and healthy dinner meal for you. This meal will be great for family and friends as well.

Serves: 4 persons
Preparation Time: 15 minutes
Cooking Time: 22 minutes

Ingredients:

- 4 (6-ounce) (1-inch thick) skinless salmon fillets
- Salt and freshly ground black pepper, to taste
- 1 (2¼-ounce) can sliced ripe olives, drained
- ½ cup zucchini, chopped finely
- 2 cups cherry tomatoes, halved
- 2 tablespoons canned capers with liquid
- 1 tablespoon olive oil

Directions:

1. Preheat the oven to 425 degrees F. Grease an 11x7-inch baking dish.
2. In a bowl, place salmon fillets and sprinkle with salt and black pepper generously.
3. Place the salmon fillets in prepared baking dish in a single layer.
4. In a bowl, mix together remaining ingredients.

5. Place the mixture over salmon fillets evenly.
6. Bake for about 22 minutes.

Nutritional Information per Serving:

Calories: 369
Fat: 23.5g
Carbohydrates: 5.2g
Dietary Fiber: 1.9g
Protein: 34.4g

Mussels in Wine & Tomato Sauce

A mouthwatering recipe of muscles... This recipe is wonderful choice for dinner from rich variety of delicious and fresh seafood... This dish is packed with sweet, spicy and tangy flavors at the same time.

Serves: 6 persons
Preparation Time: 15 minutes
Cooking Time: 20 minutes

Ingredients:

- 1 tablespoon olive oil
- 2 celery stalks, chopped
- 1 onion, chopped

- 4 garlic cloves, minced
- ½ teaspoon dried oregano, crushed
- 1 (15-ounce) can tomatoes, chopped
- 1 teaspoon honey
- 1 teaspoon red pepper flakes, crushed
- 2 pounds mussels, cleaned
- 2 cups white wine
- Salt and freshly ground black pepper, to taste
- ¼ cup fresh basil, chopped

Directions:

1. In a skillet, heat oil on medium heat.
2. Add celery, onion and garlic and sauté for about 5 minutes.
3. Add tomato, honey and red pepper flakes and simmer for about 10 minutes.
4. Meanwhile in a large pan, add mussels and wine and bring to a boil.
5. Simmer, covered for about 10 minutes.

6. Transfer the mussel mixture into tomato mixture and stir to combine.
7. Season with salt and black pepper and remove from heat.
8. Serve hot with the garnishing of basil.

Nutritional Information per Serving:

Calories: 244
Fat: 6g
Carbohydrates: 14.3g
Dietary Fiber: 1.5g
Protein: 19.1g

Lamb Chops with Herbed Pistachios

One of the super quick and simplest recipe for dinner…It is packed with wonderfully satisfying flavor of lamb with spices. Mixture of pistachio and herbs adds a flavorful richness in chops.

Serves: 4 persons
Preparation Time: 15 minutes
Cooking Time: 8 minutes

Ingredients:

For Chops:

- ½ teaspoon ground coriander
- ½ teaspoon ground cumin
- 1/8 teaspoon ground cinnamon
- Salt and freshly ground black pepper, to taste
- 8 (4-ounce) lamb loin chops, trimmed
- 1 tablespoon olive oil

For Pistachio Topping:

- 2 tablespoons pistachios, chopped finely
- 1 garlic clove, minced
- 2 teaspoons fresh lemon peel, grated finely
- 1½ tablespoons fresh cilantro, chopped
- 1½ tablespoons fresh parsley, chopped
- Salt, to taste

Directions:

1. In a large bowl, mix together spices.
2. Add lamb chops and coat with spice mixture generously.

3. In a large skillet, heat oil medium-high heat.
4. Add chops and sear for about 4 minutes per side or till desired doneness.
5. Meanwhile for topping in a bowl, mix together all ingredients.
6. Serve the chops with the topping of pistachio mixture.

Nutritional Information per Serving:

Calories: 465
Fat: 21.1g
Carbohydrates: 1.2g
Dietary Fiber: 0g
Protein: 64.2g

Lamb Kofta with Spicy Yogurt Sauce

These quick and easy lamb Kaftan patties are packed with a punch of spicy flavors. Surely this dish will satisfy your taste buds nicely. Spicy yogurt sauce pairs greatly with lamb kofta.

Serves: 6 persons
Preparation Time: 15 minutes
Cooking Time: 10 minutes

Ingredients:

For Lamb Kofta:

- 1 pound ground lamb
- 2 tablespoons fat-free plain Greek yogurt
- 2 tablespoons onion, grated
- 2 teaspoons garlic, minced
- 2 tablespoons fresh cilantro, minced
- 1 teaspoon ground coriander
- 1 teaspoon ground cumin
- 1 teaspoon ground turmeric
- Salt and freshly ground black pepper, to taste
- 1 tablespoon olive oil

For Spicy Yogurt Sauce:

- ½ cup fat-free plain Greek yogurt
- ¼ cup roasted red bell pepper, chopped

- 2 teaspoons garlic, minced
- 1 teaspoon ground coriander
- 1 teaspoon ground cumin
- ½ teaspoon red pepper flakes, crushed
- Salt, to taste

Directions:

1. For Kofta in a large bowl, add all ingredients except lamb and mix till well combined.
2. Make 12 equal sized oblong patties.
3. In a large nonstick skillet, heat oil medium-high heat.
4. Add patties and cook, flipping occasionally for about 10 minutes or till browned from both sides.
5. Meanwhile for sauce in a bowl, mix together all ingredients.
6. Serve the Kofta with the yogurt sauce.

Nutritional Information per Serving:

Calories: 185
Fat: 8.2g

Carbohydrates: 2.8g
Dietary Fiber: 0g
Protein: 24.1g

Chicken with Capers Sauce

A recipe of pan seared crispy chicken pieces with a versatile capers sauce… Coating of egg and then breadcrumb adds crispiness in chicken. The versatile capers sauce feature bold and memorable flavors.

Serves: 4 persons
Preparation Time: 15 minutes
Cooking Time: 17 minutes

Ingredients:

For Chicken:

- 2 eggs
- Salt and freshly ground black pepper, to taste
- 1 cup dry bread crumbs
- 2 tablespoons olive oil

- 1½ pound skinless, boneless chicken breast halves, pounded into ¾-inch thickness and cut into pieces

For Capers Sauce

- 3 tablespoons capers
- ½ cup dry white wine
- 3 tablespoons fresh lemon juice
- Salt and freshly ground black pepper, to taste
- 2 tablespoons fresh parsley, chopped

Directions:

1. In a shallow dish, add eggs, salt and black pepper and beat till well combined.
2. In another shallow dish, place breadcrumbs.
3. In a large skillet, heat oil on medium heat.
4. Dip the chicken pieces in egg mixture then roll in breadcrumbs evenly.
5. Shake off excess breadcrumbs

6. Add chicken in the skillet and cook for about 5-7 minutes per side or till desired doneness.
7. Transfer the chicken pieces into a plate and cover with a foil paper to keep them warm.
8. In the same skillet, add all sauce ingredients except parsley and cook, stirring for about 2-3 minutes.
9. Stir in parsley and remove from heat.
10. Serve the chicken with the topping of capers sauce.

Nutritional Information per Serving:

Calories:440
Fat:16.9g
Carbohydrates: 21.1g
Dietary Fiber: 1.5g
Protein:44.7g

Steak with Yogurt Sauce

A delicious and healthy dish... This recipe makes a great dish for family and friend's gathering for barbecue parties... This dish features grilled flank steak with refreshingly tangy Greek yogurt sauce.

Serves: 6 persons
Preparation Time: 15 minutes
Cooking Time: 12-15 minutes

Ingredients:

For Steak:

- 3 garlic cloves, minced
- 2 tablespoons fresh rosemary, chopped
- Salt and freshly ground black pepper, to taste
- 2 pounds flank steak, trimmed

For Sauce:

- 1½ cups fat-free plain Greek yogurt
- 1 cucumber, peeled, seeded and chopped finely
- 1 cup fresh parsley, chopped
- 1 garlic clove, minced
- 1 teaspoon fresh lemon zest, grated finely
- 1/8 teaspoon cayenne pepper

- Salt and freshly ground black pepper, to taste

Directions:

1. Preheat the grill to medium-high heat. Grease the grill grate.
2. For steak in a large bowl, mix together all ingredients except steak.
3. Coat the steak with mixture generously.
4. Keep aside for about 15 minutes.
5. Grill the steak for about 12-15 minutes, flipping after every 3-4 minutes.
6. Transfer the steak onto cutting board and keep aside for about 5 minutes.
7. Meanwhile for sauce in a bowl, mix together all ingredients.
8. With a sharp knife, cut the steak into desired slices.
9. Serve with the topping of yogurt sauce.

Nutritional Information per Serving:

Calories: 346
Fat: 13g

Carbohydrates: 6.4g
Dietary Fiber: 1.1g
Protein: 48.9g

Pasta with Veggies

A great addition in dinner menu list... This recipe makes a delicious dish that is a full meal too. Prepare this dish for family dinner and definitely all people would love to enjoy it.

Serves: 6 persons
Preparation Time: 15 minutes
Cooking Time: 15 minutes

Ingredients:

- 3 tomatoes
- 1 pound farfalle pasta
- ¼ cup olive oil
- 1 pound fresh mushrooms, sliced
- 3 garlic cloves, minced
- 1 teaspoondried oregano, crushed
- 1 (2-ounce) can black olives, drained
- ¾ cup feta cheese, crumbled

Directions:

1. In a large pan of salted boiling water, add tomatoes and cook for about 1 minute.
2. With a slotted spoon, transfer the tomatoes into a bowl of chilled water.
3. In the pan of boiling eater, add pasta and cook for about 8-10 minutes. Drain well.
4. Meanwhile, peel the blanched tomatoes and then chop them.
5. In a large skillet, heat oil on medium heat.
6. Add mushrooms and garlic and sauté for about 4-5 minutes.
7. Add tomatoes and oregano and cook for about 3-4 minutes.
8. Divide the pasta into serving plates and top with mushroom mixture.
9. Garnish with olives and feta and serve.

Nutritional Information per Serving:

Calories: 443
Fat: 16.5g
Carbohydrates: 57.6g
Dietary Fiber: 1.9g
Protein: 19.1g

Conclusion

It is my sincere hope that you might have liked all the recipes which have been mentioned in the book and once again thank you for getting this book and experimenting with the recipes.

About The Author

Somerville Jacques is born with the vision to promote *Mediterranean diet* among the masses. The author has written several research papers on the topic. He has served as an instructor promoting various cultural arts in University of San Francisco. He is currently living with his spouse in Texas.

www.ingramcontent.com/pod-product-compliance
Lightning Source LLC
LaVergne TN
LVHW011948070526
838202LV00054B/4846